THE
PCOS
HANDBOOK

A Comprehensive Guide to Naturally Managing
Polycystic Ovary Syndrome through Weight Loss,
Stress Management, Hormonal Balance, and
Boosting Fertility

by

W. Raymond

Table of Contents

Introduction

PCOS throwing you for a loop? Perhaps you or a loved one recently received a diagnosis of PCOS. If you want factual information about the topic, you have stopped at the right page!

This book will explore managing PCOS with minimal changes to lifestyle, diet, or overall outlook on life. Many people do not take PCOS seriously. They think it will just bar the woman from having kids, and that's it. But it's not true. We will explore this topic further in the book, but before reaching there, I want you to keep your preconceived notions to the side. Having the wrong idea is worse than having no idea.

You can truly understand and implement ways of managing PCOS if you are ready to explore practical strategies for reducing stress, eating right, exercising daily, and keeping your hormones under strict control. These natural management techniques are all you need to stay fit and fine.

As a practicing gynecologist, I have seen many distraught women find their way through life—some with enthusiasm, some with reluctance. No woman wants to go through a nerve-wreaking period such as a PCOS diagnosis, especially those who want to be mothers in the future. But with this handbook, you can expect to come to terms with the verdict and do your best to live the life you always wanted to have.

I suggest my patients adhere to the saying, *"This too shall pass."* It gives them the courage to take one step at a time and straighten out their priorities in life. You can also do the same by finding out your priorities and working towards achieving them with all your heart through this book.

Let's get started and see what PCOS is all about!

Becoming Familiar with PCOS 1

PCOS stands for Polycystic Ovary Syndrome, which affects the reproductive health of women. It causes the ovaries to have abnormal cysts in them that create complications in the regular menstruation cycle, as well as a few other factors that are vital in conceiving a child. PCOS is a hormonal condition that happens when the hormone levels are all in disarray.

It is a life-long condition that does not heal, but with a few lifestyle modifications, it is possible to live a great and fulfilling life by managing this condition. You can improve the quality of your life by exploring the ways of living that are fruitful for you.

In this chapter, we will discuss PCOS in detail. We will delve further into its symptoms, types, diagnosis, causes, risk factors, and its impact on the women's health.

1.1 What is PCOS?

Polycystic Ovary Syndrome is the excess of male hormones (androgens) and insulin in females. It happens when a woman's body produces more hormones than necessary, affecting one or both ovaries.

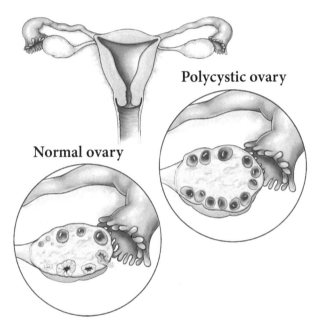

When ovaries are affected by PCOS, they form a fluid-filled sac over the immature eggs. It does not happen in every case, but it is a fairly common side effect that reduces fertility in women. These cysts are not painful or bring any further damage to the body.

PCOS can happen at any time after a girl hits puberty. Most women discover they have PCOS when they start trying for a baby in their 20s or 30s. It increases the chances of having PCOS if someone in the family has PCOS or if a woman is overweight.

PCOS and PCOD Co-Relation

You may have heard about the term PCOD (Polycystic Ovary Disease) being used as a synonym for PCOS. PCOS and PCOD are indeed very similar. They both affect the ovaries but in different capacities.

In PCOD, the ovaries are at fault for releasing eggs immaturely. It causes the ovaries to swell and create hormonal imbalances in the body. Meanwhile, PCOS is an endocrine issue that leads the ovaries to produce more androgens in the body than the necessary amount. It causes the eggs to become cysts themselves. It is also the main reason why women with PCOS have reduced chances of fertility in them, making it difficult for them to bear children despite trying.

Another glaring difference between PCOD and PCOS is that PCOD is a treatable disease, while PCOS does not go away with treatment. For both of these issues, management is vital. You can keep living the best life if you stay on top of all healthy practices.

Other Myths Regarding PCOS

Some of the other misconceptions that have taken the shape of myths are as follows:

- One cannot get pregnant with PCOS.

- One only needs to treat PCOS for pregnancy-related issues.
- If you do not have acne or hair thinning, it is not PCOS.
- Surgery is necessary for treating cysts.

All of these misconceptions are simply myths. They do not represent the facts. Some factual information is as follows:

- You can get pregnant with PCOS under special circumstances. It is not uncommon for PCOS patients to have enough fertility to bear children. It depends on each woman and her unique condition.

- As far as the treatment is concerned, you need to modify your lifestyle to stay fit. Otherwise, you are at risk for many other diseases.

- It is unlikely that a patient faces all symptoms simultaneously. If other symptoms are present, it is possible not to experience one or more symptoms completely.

- Surgery is not the solution to all problems. Cysts can re-occur, making it an unviable solution in most cases. They are also not large cysts that occur in other parts of the body, making it unrealistic to operate on them.

PCOS is a condition that has some common while other unique markers or symptoms. While there might be some myths surrounding it, you need to sift through the misconceptions to find the truth yourself. You can do so by identifying the issues and getting help from the professionals.

1.2 Symptoms and Diagnosis

There are a few indicators that hint toward some ailment in the body. PCOS has very distinct symptoms to look out for. If you feel that even half of these symptoms fit your current state, it is best to have a check-up. The main symptoms of PCOS are as follows:

- Weight Gain
- Irregular Periods
- Acne
- Abnormal Growth of Hair
- Infertility or Reduced Fertility
- Sleep Apnea
- Hair Thinning
- Darkening Skin Patches
- Cysts in Ovaries
- Skin Tags
- Pelvic Pain

These are some of the glaring symptoms that indicate the presence of PCOS in a woman's body. However, these symptoms are the first step that should always lead you to a doctor. Going there at the right time can help you in diagnosing the symptoms. It is better to be aware of your issues at the right time when minimal intervention will keep you fit and healthy.

There is no set number or order of tests that a doctor does for PCOS. They may ask you to perform any of these given tests according to your symptoms or general condition:

- **Ultrasound:** It looks for any visual changes in the ovaries or uterine lining.

- **Pelvic Exam:** This checks for growth or masses in the reproductive system and any distinctive changes in it.

- **Blood Test:** It shows hormonal changes in the body. General or targeted testing confirms the diagnosis of PCOS or any other condition mimicking its presence.

For symptoms or related issues of acne, hair loss, depression, anxiety, sleep apnea, diabetes, or high blood pressure, a doctor may suggest other tests. These related conditions may need treatment separately in the form of medications.

For PCOS itself, most women are given oral contraceptives or birth control pills to stabilize the menstruation cycle and improve other adverse effects on the body.

Types of PCOS

Every woman faces different issues due to PCOS. Some suffer from irregular periods, while others face hair loss. The difference in symptoms indicates different types of PCOS that can affect you.

They are as follows:

- Insulin Resistance PCOS
- Adrenal PCOS
- Inflammatory PCOS
- Post Pill PCOS

1. Insulin Resistance PCOS

It is the most common type of PCOS. It occurs when the body's insulin starts losing its effectiveness. It increases fatigue, sugar cravings, and weight in the abdominal area.

A balanced diet, proper sleep, and controlled stress levels can help manage insulin levels. Regular exercise can keep the harmful effects of PCOS away from the body.

2. Adrenal PCOS

This type of PCOS occurs when you are going through a stressful time in your life. In this state, Dehydroepiandrosterone (DHEA) and cortisol shoot up, indicating the presence of adrenal PCOS.

With this type of PCOS, high-intensity exercises are not recommended. You can do meditation or yoga, which reduces extreme stress.

3. Inflammatory PCOS

Inflammatory PCOS occurs when you face chronic inflammation. An unhealthy lifestyle and diet cause an increase in testosterone levels, which leads to PCOS. It causes skin issues, headaches, high C reactive proteins, or unexplained fatigue.

Taking natural anti-inflammatory foods or manufactured medications can help manage the condition and maintain gut health.

4. Post-Pill PCOS

Most women are given contraceptive pills as a treatment for PCOS. It keeps the body regularized with its intake but creates an issue when you stop the pills. The controlled symptoms can get worse after stopping the intake.

The good news is that it is a reversible condition that happens temporarily. Keeping your lifestyle and diet in check can help you eradicate it easily.

These conditions are often supplemented with nutrients (natural or artificial) that doctors prescribe after a detailed check-up. You can also manage your PCOS type by taking a proper diet and taking care of yourself physically, mentally, and emotionally.

1.3 Causes and Risk Factors

There are only speculations about the causes of PCOS at this point. There are some guesses as to what causes a body to develop PCOS, but the real reasons are not yet introduced conclusively.

Your family history is likely to increase your level of risk. Genetics, environmental factors, and lifestyle are other possibilities currently under study.

You increase the risk of developing other health conditions if you do not care for your nutritional health. Diabetes, high blood pressure, chances of stroke, high cholesterol, abnormalities in lipid profile, and other such conditions develop with negligence and inattentiveness to health.

One symptom and risk factor for PCOS is the development of sleep apnea. It is the sudden inability to breathe while sleeping. It is a severe condition that can even lead to death in rare cases. Sleep apnea can cause a person to feel sleepy and tired throughout the day because of disturbed sleep at night.

Another risk that occurs in extreme cases is no ovulation. When you do not ovulate regularly, the lining of the uterus does not shed away. This increases the chance of endometrial cancer, among other issues.

Who Gets It?

Almost 5-10% of women, after reaching the age of puberty, can be diagnosed with PCOS. There is no classification of who can get it, but most women get to know they have PCOS when they seek treatment for getting pregnant.

1.4 Impact on Women's Health

Women's health can have long-lasting impact because of PCOS. When you get to know about your diagnosis, many thoughts and ideas start circling in your mind. Sometimes, it's about your future and health complications that can arise later; other times, it's about your ability to start a family.

Some women worry themselves to the point of being sick, while others start taking measures aggressively. There are very limited options for you to choose from after a diagnosis. Even if you feel bothered, managing all issues is better than giving up.

Short-Term and Long-Term Health Implications

If you know the implications of a condition, you can expand your knowledge base and take effective measures. This can only happen if you stay informed about ever-evolving research and find the best solutions for yourself.

Some short-term consequences of getting PCOS are as follows:

- Increases Menstrual Irregularities.
- Creates Hormonal Imbalance.
- Raises Metabolic Issues.
- Increases Psychological Pressure.

Some long-term implications of having PCOS are as follows:

- Increases Risk of Cardiovascular Diseases.
- Increases Risk of Diabetes.
- Increases Risk of Getting Obese.
- Increases Risk of Endometrial Cancer.
- Increases Risk of Infertility Issues.

Health implications come with each issue. No disease or condition stays separated from the rest of the body. It affects every woman differently.

Emotional and Psychological Effects

Nothing in our life happens without making us feel some psychological or emotional effects. It can simply be a painful moment you want to move on from or a long-term struggle that takes time to come to terms with. All of your feelings are validated. You can feel as you please; just try to listen to your own struggles and face them with a brave face on.

A few of those common struggles are mentioned ahead that women with PCOS complain about the most. They are given here:

Issues with Body Image

When a woman starts gaining weight, she is likelier to feel insecure about her physical appearance. It makes her feel judged and less appreciated for the other qualities that are worthy of praise. Their self-perception takes a severe hit, especially for women with facial hair growth.

Impact on Daily Life

Usually, when women find out about their PCOS, they are already overweight. It means that their daily lives require a balanced diet, exercise, stress control, and other measures that make them feel more pressured.

Please note here that not all women get obese with PCOS, but most of them do.

A woman goes through stages of grief that result in her lethargic and stressed state of mind. Some women develop depression or anxiety because of not being able to cope with the diagnosis.

Issues with Sexual Life

Most PCOS patients are dissatisfied with their sexual lives because of several issues occurring in their ability to feel pleasure. Having infertility is an issue for some, but all patients report their insecurities about body image, unusual hair growth, and other such things disrupting the forming of lasting connections with other people especially with their spouses.

These are some of the impacting factors of a PCOS diagnosis that become a point of friction in most cases. You need lasting satisfaction to be yourself and happy, but it can only happen when you are ready to let the impact not disturb your peace of mind.

The Role of Diet and Nutrition 2

Hormonal and other relevant issues of PCOS can be managed with proper intake of diet and nutrition. It is important in daily life for many reasons, which will be discussed in detail later.

It is important to learn the art of making plates to maintain a good diet. Yes, we need to include and exclude certain items from the diet. But you need to learn the most basic lesson there is: the quantities of portions.

We all know that we need to include proteins, vegetables, healthy fats, and fruits in our diet. Focusing on HOW to eat right can make you more conscious of your eating habits, no matter where you are.

Even if you are on vacation, visiting family, or on a business trip, you can eat the right things at the right time without depending on others to point out certain foods.

When making a plate, it should include:

- ¼ plate of protein (25-30 grams)
- ½ plate of non-starchy vegetables
- ¼ plate of starchy vegetables or legumes

It makes a complete plate for a balanced meal. It should look like this:

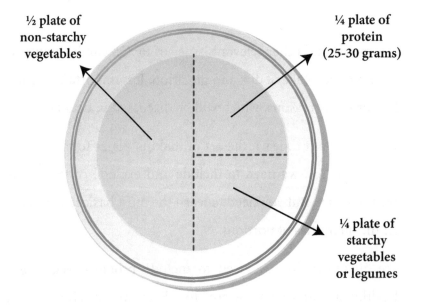

½ plate of non-starchy vegetables

¼ plate of protein (25-30 grams)

¼ plate of starchy vegetables or legumes

When setting a plate, you need protein in the form of chicken, fish, or meat for a non-vegetarian diet and lentils, nuts, quinoa, oats, or beans for a vegetarian diet.

Nuts and seeds can help add healthy fats to the plate. Olive oil, roasted vegetables, and olives are other options.

For non-starchy vegetables, you need broccoli, cauliflower, tomatoes, mushrooms, leafy greens, radishes, and eggplants, among others. For starchy vegetables and legumes, you have options from brown rice, whole-grain bread, corn, beets, sweet potatoes, etc.

2.1 The PCOS-Friendly Diet

A PCOS-friendly diet does not mean that you need to follow a dash diet that overcomplicates your daily management. Don't get me wrong; it does not mean that all diets are like that. But we must understand that consuming healthy food is not a "trend" that should be changed with the wind; instead, it is a lifestyle you must choose for yourself at the right time.

If you feel that some diet can positively change your life, go for it. But focus on rules rather than recipes. If you are familiar with the intake rules, you are more likely to make the process easier on you.

If you are ready to start a balanced diet, you need to include and exclude a few items from it. They are provided ahead.

Foods to Include

The foods which you need to add to your diet are as follows:

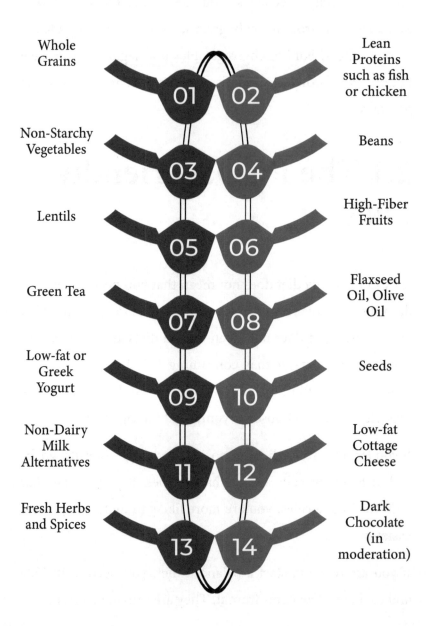

Whole Grains — 01

Lean Proteins such as fish or chicken — 02

Non-Starchy Vegetables — 03

Beans — 04

Lentils — 05

High-Fiber Fruits — 06

Green Tea — 07

Flaxseed Oil, Olive Oil — 08

Low-fat or Greek Yogurt — 09

Seeds — 10

Non-Dairy Milk Alternatives — 11

Low-fat Cottage Cheese — 12

Fresh Herbs and Spices — 13

Dark Chocolate (in moderation) — 14

Foods to Avoid

The foods which you need to avoid in your diet are as follows:

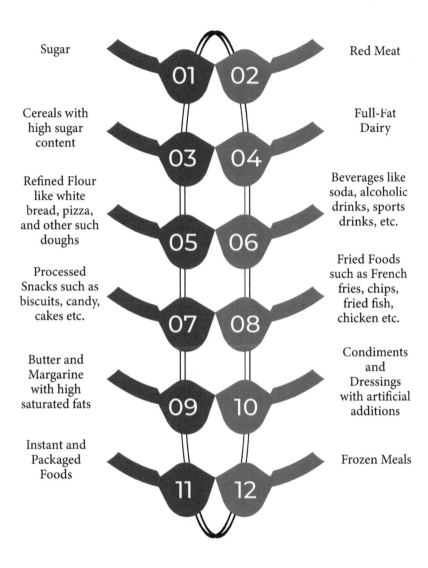

Sugar

Red Meat

Cereals with high sugar content

Full-Fat Dairy

Refined Flour like white bread, pizza, and other such doughs

Beverages like soda, alcoholic drinks, sports drinks, etc.

Processed Snacks such as biscuits, candy, cakes etc.

Fried Foods such as French fries, chips, fried fish, chicken etc.

Butter and Margarine with high saturated fats

Condiments and Dressings with artificial additions

Instant and Packaged Foods

Frozen Meals

01 02 03 04 05 06 07 08 09 10 11 12

Once you are aware of the things you need to do, you can manage yourself better for a long time. You can also create a plan to increase the nutritional value of your meals.

Benefits

PCOS diet has a few benefits that increase your chances of managing this life-long condition most optimally. Some of these benefits are as follows:

- A low-glycemic index diet can increase digestion and slow down absorption in the body. It can manage the blood sugar level along with insulin sensitivity.

- Consuming nutrients in a balanced way can increase hormonal balance in the body. Antioxidants, omega-3 fatty acids, vitamins, and minerals are all essential for a body.

- It also helps with weight management. You can stay within the recommended weight frame through portion control and healthy intake.

- A PCOS-friendly diet also allows the body to have good reproductive health. It naturally provides you with folate, iron, and other nutrients necessary for the body's reproductive functions.

- Inflammation can exacerbate the PCOS. Using anti-inflammatory foods in the diet allows you to keep such complications at bay or even treat them better.

These are some of the basic benefits that PCOS-friendly food can provide you. It is better to know which items are necessary and what to use. Moderation is the key here.

2.2 Essential Nutrients for Balancing Hormones

Hormones are never stable in a woman's body. Due to menstruation and other changes, they keep going up and down. When it comes to PCOS, the irregularities in your period can cause you to have an upheaval in the body that results in hormonal imbalance eventually.

Nutrients are essential for all parts of the body to perform their best. When trying to entertain the essential ones, you may need help from natural or artificial resources to find the best solution. It is crucial to know why these nutrients are considered necessary and what you need to look for while buying them.

Role of Vitamins, Minerals, and Antioxidants

Vitamins and minerals are important for the normal functioning of the body. They help support growth, boost the immune system, fight infections, regulate hormones, make bones strong, and heal wounds.

Antioxidants are also responsible for healing wounds and destroying the "free radicals" compound, which damages cell membranes.

Commonly Recommended Supplements

PCOS is a condition closely linked to many nutrient deficiencies. Most women face disturbances in one or more basic nutrients that are required for optimal daily body functioning.

The supplements are all the extra help you can get from external sources for your health. If your body develops a deficiency, it is better to get help from supplements rather than natural sources like fruits and vegetables.

The most common supplements that you may require are as follows:

- Vitamin C
- Vitamin D
- B Vitamins (B6, B12)
- Omega-3
- Magnesium

It is to be noted here that these supplements are not for everyday usage unless a doctor advises you to use them. PCOS can cause a deficiency of any vitamin or mineral, common or uncommon, that requires intervention from you and your doctor.

Mcrits for Choosing Quality Supplements

When choosing supplements, a few parameters must be kept in check. There are too many options available in the market, some of which may or may not be of good quality.

If you want to buy the supplements, choose one that holds the given merits. They are as follows:

1. **Independent Third Party Tested:** If the independent third party tests a supplement, it means that the quality check results are unbiased and completely reliable.

2. **Pharmaceutical Grade:** When a supplement is a pharmaceutical grade, the chemicals and methods used in its making ensure maximum benefit to the patient. There are no fillers or unusable ingredients in their making.

3. **Chelated Minerals:** These are minerals that are chemically combined with amino acids. Amino acids help with faster absorption of these minerals and ensure the bioavailability of the used ingredients.

When you are buying supplements for yourself or family members, make sure to take these merits into account.

2.3 Meal Planning and Ideas

Meals seem boring when you can't think of making something tasty to eat. With PCOS and other conditions that require lifestyle modifications, you need to devise enough variations and routines to keep food-making and eating interesting.

The recipes and sample planner in this section will help you prepare great recipes and get new ideas for a balanced diet.

Recipes for PCOS

Here are some recipes you can use to experiment with new flavors and ingredients that are good for your PCOS-friendly diet.

Baked Granola

Serves 6

Ingredients

Almonds	1/2 cup
Walnuts	1/2 cup
Pecans	1/2 cup
Apples (grated)	1 tbsp.
Flaxseed	2 tbsp.

Coconut flakes	1/3 cup
Almond Milk	1/2 cup
Coconut Oil	3 tbsp. (1 tbsp. for toasting nuts, 2 tbsp. for granola mixture)
Apple Pie Spice	1 tbsp.
Ground Ceylon Cinnamon	1 tsp.
Salt	1/2 tsp.
Water	5 tbsp.

Instructions

1. Put the flaxseeds in water and set them aside to thicken for approximately 15 minutes.

2. Preheat the oven to 350 °F.

3. Prepare the baking sheet by lining it with parchment paper.

4. Add all the nuts and coconut flakes to the sheet and drizzle with coconut oil. Roast for 5 minutes, then take it out of the oven and cool it down.

5. Set the oven temperature to 375°F.

6. In a food processor, pulse the roasted nuts until they crumble into chunks, but do not over grind them.

7. Mix the roughly ground nuts and strained flaxseed in a big bowl with all other ingredients.

8. Transfer the mixture to a 9" x 9" baking dish and bake for 35 to 40 minutes. It should look brown and crispy on top after this time.

Feta and Chicken Pasta

Serves 4

Ingredients

Chicken Breast	1/2 lb.
Feta Cheese	8 oz.
Chickpea Pasta	8 oz.
Cherry Tomatoes	2 pints
Baby Spinach	2 cups
Garlic Cloves (minced)	5
Basil (chopped)	1/4 cup
Salt	1/4 tsp.
Black Pepper	1/4 tsp.
Olive Oil	1/3 cup

Instructions

1. Preheat the oven to 400 °F.

2. Take a 9" x 13" baking dish and place the chicken breast and a block of cheese into it. Add cherry tomatoes, garlic, olive oil, salt, and pepper into the dish and toss the ingredients.

3. Put it in the oven for 35 minutes once the ingredients are adequately coated.

4. Make the chickpea pasta according to the package instructions.

5. Once cooked, remove the chicken, cut it into pieces, and put it aside.

6. Now, mash the tomatoes and cheese with the spoon and put the dish back inside.

7. Take the dish out again and add basil, spinach, and chicken while stirring the mixture gently. The spinach should wilt after some stirring.

8. Add the pasta and combine it well. You can also garnish it with Parmesan cheese.

Salmon Salad

Ingredients

Baked Salmon	8 oz.
Mixed Greens	2 cups
Radishes (sliced)	4
Mint	1/4 cup
Green Onions (thinly sliced)	2
Strawberries	1 & 1/2 cup
Pumpkin Seeds (toasted)	1/4 cup
Extra Virgin Olive Oil	2 tbsp.
Balsamic Glaze	2 tsp.
Goat Cheese	2 oz. (optional)
Salt	to taste
Black Pepper	to taste

Instructions

1. Mix the greens with salt, pepper, and oil in a big bowl. After tossing, divide them into two bowls.

2. Add the Salmon, radishes, mint, strawberries, green onions, pumpkin seeds, and goat cheese to both bowls.

3. Drizzle the balsamic glaze over bowls before serving the salad.

Pineapple Mocktail

Serves 2

Ingredients

Pineapple (cubed)	1 cup
Lime (juiced)	2
Coconut Water	1 & 1/2 cup
Monkfruit Sweetener	1 tsp.
Sea Salt	1/2 tsp.

Instructions

1. Add all ingredients in a blender and blend for 30 seconds.
2. Pour the prepared mocktails into glasses (with or without ice) as you prefer.

Shrimp Fried Rice

Serves 4

Ingredients

Shrimps (peeled and deveined)	20 oz.
Mushrooms (finely diced)	2 cups

Zucchini (finely diced)	1
Carrots (finely diced)	2
Onion (finely diced)	1
Scallions (chopped)	4
Garlic (minced)	2 tsp.
Cauliflower (riced)	6 cups
Gluten-free Tamari Sauce	3 tbsp.
Coconut Aminos	3 tbsp.
Fish Sauce	1 tbsp.
Coconut Oil	2 tbsp.
Salt	1/4 tsp.

Instructions

1. Heat the oil over medium heat and cook the shrimp for 5 minutes.

2. Set the shrimp aside. Meanwhile, cook the carrots, zucchini, mushrooms, onion, and garlic for 5 minutes while stirring occasionally.

3. Now, remove the vegetables and cook the cauliflower for 5 minutes. If it dries up, add more coconut oil.

4. Add the shrimp and vegetables back to the pan along with

the tamari sauce, coconut aminos, and fish sauce. Stir and cook for 2 minutes.

5. Season it with salt and add scallions as a garnish.

Note:

Shrimp Fried Rice can be stored in an airtight container for up to 3 days in the refrigerator.

Fajita Steak

Serves 4

Ingredients

Flank Steak (sliced into 1/4 inches strips against the grain)	2 lbs.
Flour or Corn Tortillas	8
Bell Peppers	4
Garlic Cloves (minced)	2
Medium-Sized Yellow Onion (sliced)	1
Fresh Lime (juiced)	2
Chili Powder	1 tbsp.
Garlic Powder	1 tsp.
Black Pepper	1/2 tsp.

Ground Cumin	1 tsp.
Paprika	1/2 tsp.
Sea Salt	1/2 tsp.
Olive Oil	2 tbsp.

Optional Topping

- Guacamole
- Mexican Cheese Blend
- Cilantro
- Lime Juice
- Sliced Avocado
- Diced Tomatoes

Instructions

1. Preheat the oven to 400 °F.

2. Spray the non-stick oil on a large baking pan or foil it.

3. Mix the chili powder, sea salt, cumin, black pepper, and garlic in a bowl to make fajita seasoning and set aside.

4. Now, put the steak slices in a zip-lock bag and add the juice of one lime, one tbsp. of olive oil, and two-thirds of the seasoning you just made. Lock the bag and mix it until the steak is fully coated. Put it in the fridge for at least 15 minutes (preferably overnight).

5. Place the sliced onion and bell peppers on the baking sheet, along with the remaining olive oil and seasoning. Toss the ingredients.

6. Bake it in the oven for 15 minutes before pulling it out and making room for the steak slices.

7. Put the steak on the same sheet, maintaining an even layer of all ingredients, and cook for another 10 to 12 minutes. You can also cook the steak according to your preference.

8. Warm the tortillas before adding all the ingredients. Top them with lime juice, paprika, or any number of toppings. The quantity and toppings can be adjusted according to taste and choice.

Mango Smoothie

Serves 2

Ingredients

Frozen Mango	3 cups
Protein Powder	3 tbsp.
Almond Milk (unsweetened)	1/2 cup
Coconut Milk (unsweetened)	1/2 cup
Greek Yogurt	1/2 cup
Flaxseed (grounded)	2 tbsp.

Instructions

1. Add all ingredients in a blender and blend for 30 seconds or more.

2. Once it reaches smoothness in texture, it is ready to drink.

Sample Meal Plan

Making a meal plan can be very hectic and frustrating when you are out of ideas or need an urgent fix. You can make a plan similar to the one here by incorporating your favorites.

I have left the given recipes for you to incorporate in your planner, not the ones given here. This will increase the number of options you have to choose from.

	Day 1	Day 2	Day 3
Breakfast	Greek yogurt with a handful of berries and a tablespoon of chia seeds	Overnight oats made with almond milk, topped with sliced banana and a sprinkle of flaxseeds	Smoothie with spinach, frozen berries, half a banana, and unsweetened almond milk
	Green tea	Herbal tea	A boiled egg
Mid-Morning Snack	A small apple with a tablespoon of almond butter	A pear	Sliced cucumber with guacamole
Lunch	Grilled chicken salad with mixed greens, cherry tomatoes, cucumber, avocado, and a light vinaigrette dressing	Quinoa and black bean bowl with corn, bell peppers, avocado, and a squeeze of lime	Turkey and avocado wrap in a whole grain tortilla with a side salad
	Whole grain crackers	A side of mixed greens	-

	Day 1	Day 2	Day 3
Afternoon Snack	Carrot sticks with hummus	A handful of berries	A handful of almonds
Dinner	Baked salmon with a side of quinoa and steamed broccoli	Stir-fried tofu with mixed vegetables (broccoli, bell peppers, snap peas) in a light soy-ginger sauce	Baked chicken breast with sweet potato wedges and sautéed green beans
	Mixed green salad with olive oil and lemon dressing	Brown rice	Mixed green salad with balsamic vinaigrette
Supper	A small bowl of mixed nuts (unsalted)	Greek yogurt with a drizzle of honey	A small bowl of cottage cheese with pineapple chunks

	Day 4	Day 5	Day 6	Day 7
Breakfast	Scrambled eggs with spinach and tomatoes, A slice of whole grain toast	Chia seed pudding made with coconut milk, topped with fresh mango and a sprinkle of coconut flakes	Smoothie bowl with spinach, frozen berries, a scoop of protein powder, and topped with granola and chia seeds	Greek yogurt parfait with layers of mixed berries, granola, and a drizzle of honey
	Herbal tea	Green tea	Herbal tea	Green tea
Mid-Morning Snack	A peach	An orange	A small bowl of strawberries	A kiwi
Lunch	Lentil soup with a side of whole grain bread	Chickpea and avocado salad with cherry tomatoes, cucumber, red onion, and feta cheese	Grilled vegetable wrap with hummus in a whole grain tortilla	Quinoa salad with roasted vegetables (sweet potato, bell peppers, red onion) and a tahini dressing
	Carrot and celery sticks	Whole grain pita bread	Side of mixed greens	Side of mixed greens

	Day 4	Day 5	Day 6	Day 7
Afternoon Snack	A handful of walnuts	A handful of pistachios	A sliced apple with a tablespoon of peanut butter	Sliced bell peppers with hummus
Dinner	Grilled shrimp with a quinoa and vegetable stir-fry (zucchini, bell peppers, onions)	Baked cod with roasted Brussels sprouts and a side of wild rice	Turkey meatballs with zucchini noodles and marinara sauce	Grilled chicken breast with a side of brown rice and steamed broccoli
	Side salad with lemon-olive oil dressing	Mixed green salad with vinaigrette	Steamed asparagus	Mixed green salad with olive oil and lemon dressing
Supper	A small bowl of mixed berries	Greek yogurt with a handful of granola	A handful of mixed nuts (unsalted)	A small bowl of cottage cheese with a few slices of cucumber

By now, you have an idea of how meal planners work. You can make your own diet planners by following the same patterns we have used in this chapter. While making a plan, make sure to have balanced meals on a daily basis.

You may find and incorporate new recipes in your daily schedule. As long as they are healthy and balanced, you can bring innovation that can be managed from your end with ease.

Weight Loss Strategies 3

Weight loss is challenging if you do not feel motivated to take it to the end – by hook or crook. If you need to lose weight, you can implement the strategies given in this chapter to make a workout plan that works best for you.

Weight never drops down until you put effort into it. Understanding the role of increased weight in PCOS can allow you to integrate the best practices into your routine.

3.1 The Connection Between Weight and PCOS

The connection between weight and PCOS is fairly simple yet complex. Many knots in this thread have yet to be resolved. This means we do not have a clear cause for how they affect each other, but the important part is that they do have an effect on each other.

It can be taken as a cycle of effects that keep influencing the other factor: weight gain upsets PCOS, while PCOS upsets weight (increasing it because of several other factors).

When you have PCOS, you are more than likely to gain weight if you are not conscious of your diet and habits. If you simply control your portions or calories, you can lose weight. Moderate exercise is the best way to maintain your weight and figure without much intervention.

By controlling your weight, you can also increase your fertility and metabolic health. A visit to a nutritionist can also help maintain the weight that causes your abdominal area to put on more than necessary.

Benefits of Weight Loss

Being overweight, you can get the benefits mentioned ahead from losing weight when you have PCOS.

- It helps your reproductive health functions, such as ovulation and regulating the menstrual cycle.

- It also contributes to helping with conceiving.

- It lessens the intensity of PCOS symptoms (but doesn't finish them altogether).

- It helps with making insulin resistance in the body.

- It helps reduce the risk of other serious health issues like heart health.

When you are determined to make significant changes, it is best to start with a weight loss regimen because it has shown results in the past.

3.2 Effective Exercise Routines

Exercise is a basic need of the body. When you are ready to create a new and improved routine for yourself, you can easily achieve balance. Exercise can help increase insulin sensitivity and improve menstrual, cardiovascular, and mental health.

To positively impact life-long health, you can adjust your physical activity time to support your overall health. You can choose any type of exercise as long as it is easy and fun for you.

Types of Exercises

The exercises and their further classifications are very diverse. You can choose any type of exercise as long as it remains doable for you. It can be a challenging task to take on, especially when you have not been taking care of yourself.

Some types of exercises are as follows:

- **Aerobic Exercise** means any activity that spikes your breathing and heart rate through physical training. It can include brisk walking, running, hiking, cycling, rowing, and playing games like tennis and badminton.

- **Flexibility Exercises** include any activity that focuses on making your body more agile. Stretching, dancing, deep squats, and yoga are all recommended to increase flexibility. By working on breathing techniques along with these exercises, you can optimize the experience even more.

- **Strength Training** focuses on strengthening your muscles and bones and improving your posture. Some exercises you can use for it are Pilates, weight lifting, push-ups, lunges, and exercises with a resistance band.

You can use these exercises to make a plan that fits your work and home routine without disturbing anything.

Creating a Balanced Workout Plan

A planner for a balanced exercise routine is a must. You can make yours by following some of these valuable tips:

- Set a time limit. Make sure to ease into the routine by starting with 20 or 30 minutes and increasing the time limit as you become assimilated to it.

- Experiment with the poses and exercises. Following the routine means starting with exercises that are easy for you and gradually increasing the difficulty level.

- Include breaks and pauses. You do not need to plan and execute exercises for all seven days of the week. It can have a break after three days or so to keep the routine palatable.

- Keep a balanced routine. You cannot ruin the balance by exercising too much for a day and leaving the practice for three days in a row.

Now, keeping these tips in mind, make a planner for yourself. It should include at least three different poses/exercises for your practice. Add your time limits for each day and its division in each cell.

Days	Exercises		
Day 1			
Day 2			
Day 3			
Day 4			
Day 5			
Day 6			
Day 7			

Caution!

If you are starting out exercising out of the blue, it is better to create an easy routine first. You need to make sure that muscles are not being unnecessarily stretched. With obesity, it is easy to strain muscles if you are not careful.

3.3 Building a Sustainable Weight Loss Plan

When creating a weight loss plan, it is best to form it by adding things that ensure its sustainability and long-term engagement. If you are one of those who get bored easily, it is best to encourage yourself by using the strategies provided here:

1. Visualize the Action

When starting an exercise is difficult, it is recommended that you visualize yourself doing it. For example, cardio is a difficult exercise. While learning the exercises, you can envision yourself and the precise movements you will perform.

2. Setting Realistic Goals

When you are setting your exercise goals, keep your capability in mind. You can set competitive or challenging goals for yourself that are beyond your current capacity, but they should be realistic.

It will help you regularize your exercise routine while progressing toward your future goal of staying fit.

3. Monitoring Progress

When you constantly check your progress, you can see the difference in real-time. Small and constant changes in weight loss can also motivate you to do better and make a real difference.

4. Combine the Goals

If you have issues making and completing exercise goals, it is best to combine the goal with something from your daily routine that has become a habit at this point. For example, if you brush your teeth at night, you can combine this task with walking before or after. With just 30 minutes of walking or any other type of activity, you can stay on track.

5. Set the Mood

Using music along with the exercises can set the mood. It can help you get in the zone and work harder to lose weight. A workout playlist can bring immense motivation to the scene.

6. Pick and Choose the Moves

It is not necessary to try every exercise available on Earth. You can choose the specific poses and exercises that are easy for you and fulfill the purpose of losing weight.

These are some of the strategies that can help you build a workout plan that benefits you in the long run. Learning about the exercises or how to do them is not enough. You need to be able to show the effort required to make a real change.

Stress Management Techniques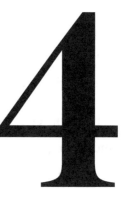

Stress reaches everyone. It does not discriminate against age, race, caste, or creed. You know what happens when a stressor starts multiplying in the head? It disturbs your whole life, keeps the gears of the head constantly running, disrupts sleep cycles, and makes it difficult to have any joys in life.

Once it starts disturbing or destroying you, you can never be at peace. However, you can slow down your incredibly stressed life by introducing some techniques we will discuss in this chapter.

4.1 How Stress Affects PCOS

Stress or any other issue that affects the body creates a chain response reaction. The body perceives a threat and takes measures. But sometimes, the body receives wrong information from its sources and takes wrong measures.

When you encounter a stress-inducing situation, it builds up and then goes away. This is acute stress. But when the constant stress persists, it develops into chronic stress, which forces the body to stay in the "fight-or-flight" zone. It creates an excess of cortisol in the body, which affects all its functions by not letting it rest.

Excessive stress in the body also increases anxiety, fatigue, headaches, digestive problems, and other such problems. PCOS in itself can work as a catalyst for inducing stress and its retention. You are six times more at risk for experiencing excessive stress and anxiety if you have PCOS.

4.2 Creating a Stress-Free Environment

A stress-free environment means changing your experience and possible ways of coping. You cannot end your worries by clapping once. There is no shortcut to staying happy and fulfilled without any stressors.

Here is what you can try to minimize the adverse effects of a stressful life:

- **Therapy:** If it is difficult to find good listeners or you struggle to come to terms with the diagnosis, you can try therapy. It will help you find healthy coping mechanisms and some emotional stability.

- **Deep Breathing Techniques:** These techniques allow you to focus on your breathing patterns to pull the mind away from stressors. They force you to relax the body, increasing its situational awareness and reducing stress.

- **Meditation:** Meditative practices are widely acclaimed for reducing stress. They allow you to clear your mind by bringing focus to the present. You can use any exercise as long as it helps you activate your imagination.

- **Self-Care Practices:** Finding time to use self-care techniques to calm down can also help you establish your resting time. If you can spend time improving your mood and listening to your own thoughts, it will help you rejuvenate yourself to face the challenges of life.

- **Mindful Movement:** Focusing on your body and its movements while performing a daily life activity such as gardening, washing dishes, cooking, etc., can reduce stress levels.

- **Getting Full Sleep:** Getting 7-9 hours of sleep keeps many stressors at bay. It helps alleviate stress and improve memory and concentration skills.

These are some of the most useful techniques for reducing stress and focusing on its positive effects in general. By making small and seemingly inconsequential changes, you can feel the difference in a stress-free life.

Balancing Hormones Naturally 5

Hormones form in all endocrine glands of the body, including the thyroid, pineal gland, adrenal gland, pituitary gland, thymus, pancreas, ovaries, and testes (only in males).

These hormones are produced in very small amounts, but they still cause significant changes in the body. If hormone production increases or decreases, it can have serious consequences.

If you are aware of how each hormone impacts your body differently, it will help you make informed decisions in the future. This chapter will educate you about hormones, their imbalance, and how you can keep them in check with useful techniques.

5.1 Understanding Hormonal Imbalances in PCOS

The hormonal imbalance is one of the critical markers of PCOS. It affects everyone at some level. When a woman goes through the symptoms of PCOS, it is likely for her to go through some unwanted changes. It is best to gain knowledge of the body's changes for proper mitigation.

Key Hormones Involved

The hormones that are disturbed because of the PCOS are as follows:

- **Testosterone** is also produced in the female body, conversely to popular opinion. However, a female body only makes a small amount of it, which rises to high levels because of PCOS.

- **Sex Hormone-Binding Globulin (SHBG)** is a protein that binds testosterone with the blood and reduces its effects. PCOS affects it by increasing its levels in the body.

- **Luteinizing Hormone (LH)** is responsible for stimulating ovulation. When it increases in PCOS to an abnormal level, it affects the ovaries.

- **Insulin** is the hormone that controls the amount of sugar in the body. Insulin resistance is an issue that increases in PCOS patients if they do not modify their lifestyle.

- **Prolactin** is a hormone responsible for producing milk in the breast gland. It increases in some women with PCOS, but not all.

These hormones are affected by the changes in a body with PCOS. It has been suggested that ovaries, responsible glands, or a part of the brain might be responsible for this imbalance, but there are no irrefutable proofs to back that claim.

How Imbalances Affect the Body

When discussing how a body is affected by these hormones, let's first understand the reproductive system. It is essential to understand how a regular menstrual cycle works and how it differs from the process in a PCOS patient's body.

The differences between the cycles of ordinary and PCOS menstruation cycle are as follows:

Normal Menstrual Cycle	PCOS-Affected Menstrual Cycle
Normal cycle ranges between 25-35 days.	Generally irregular cycles.
Follicle-making happens most optimally.	Small follicles in the ovary form cysts, reducing fertility.

Normal Menstrual Cycle	PCOS-Affected Menstrual Cycle
Average/Normal production of the follicle-stimulating hormone (FSH), LH, estrogen, and progesterone.	High production of LH and FSH, while low production of estrogen and progesterone.

These changes raise androgen levels in women. An increase in insulin is also responsible for raising androgen levels in the body.

Insulin resistance occurs when insulin is not produced in the body, while hyperinsulinemia is the excess production of insulin when it is not needed.

It is a myth that insulin resistance or hyperinsulinemia can only happen to overweight females. It is entirely false. In PCOS, you can get these complications even when you have normal weight. You are simply at an increased risk of developing severe conditions when you are overweight and not trying to maintain the weight.

5.2 Lifestyle Changes for Hormonal Health

Setting a healthy routine is essential to living a good life ahead. Your hormonal health will define your feelings and moods at any given time. These feelings will, in turn, outline how a person will behave and take action at any time. This is a cycle of how a small change can significantly impact the whole of your life.

If you need to create a working regimen of daily life ahead, you must follow some of the important factors.

Sleep and Circadian Rhythms

Your body needs rest and regulated patterns to stay healthy. With PCOS, you can experience any type of sleep disturbance or disorder. The hormonal imbalance also affects the sleep cycle, which makes it difficult for women to get quality sleep.

These disturbances further affect the metabolic rate and other linked functions of the body. Sleep disruption can create a running issue with following a diet plan and having lower energy than necessary.

You can improve your sleep by sleeping early and making the most of nighttime. Taking a nap in between day time can also help you improve your routine.

You can consult and get medication for any treatable conditions in extreme circumstances.

Reducing Exposure to Endocrine Disruptors

Endocrine disruptors are the hormones that create hormonal imbalances in the first place. We already know how these hormones create disturbances that are responsible for disruptions in daily life.

By treating the hormonal changes and monitoring them closely, you can allow the body to breathe freely and not cause issues in other activities.

Working with Healthcare Providers

The best option for any condition is to seek a doctor's opinion. When you are in close contact with your doctor, they will guide you on best practices for yourself. These could include medication, other treatment options, or lifestyle changes, but they all converge on a single goal: making your life easier.

Boosting Fertility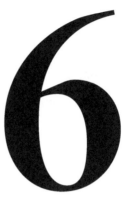

Fertility is one of the essential functions of the reproductive system. In females, it is the ability to get pregnant. An average woman in her 20s goes through the cycle with around a 25-30% chance of getting pregnant each month. This percentage gets critically low when you have PCOS.

Let's discuss how women with PCOS face challenges, available treatment options for them, and how to track ovulation.

6.1 PCOS and Fertility Challenges

In PCOS, there is more than likely a chance of women experiencing fertility issues. Understanding the stats and issues beforehand is best to prepare your mind and body for the upcoming challenges.

When PCOS is involved, getting the desired results is a factor of luck and chance. Doing everything right does not ensure anything. You may get results or not; the only thing you can do is try your best. By understanding your body better, you can increase the chances of receiving the desired results.

How PCOS Affects Ovulation

In normal circumstances, usually one egg forms in each month's cycle, but in PCOS, it either does not develop or is not released at the right time. It causes a lot of issues with fertility and subsequent pregnancy.

But there is a genuine probability that with the help of targeted medication or other methods, there is a chance of getting pregnant. Most women take time to conceive or try multiple methods to be successful. Around 30% of women with PCOS do get pregnant (with or without intervention through different available treatment options).

Common Issues with PCOS

Most women with PCOS have to face infertility. If you do not have periods, you are also free from the issues that pregnancy and its associated factors can cause. But if you have a chance of getting pregnant, however small, it is better to explore the available options thoroughly and make a sound decision about whether going for extensive treatments like IVF is beneficial for you or not. When women decide to pursue pregnancy, they are unaware of many consequences and factors. They should be aware of what they can face in the near future before making a decision.

The fertility issues that affect pregnancy with PCOS are as follows:

- Gestational Diabetes or other conditions with temporary effects
- Miscarriage
- Cesarean Section
- Preeclampsia

6.2 Course of Treatment

If PCOS makes you completely infertile, there is nothing you can do to reverse it. However, if there is even a chance of fertility, there are a few common treatments that are used. It is better to familiarize yourself with the most acceptable treatments for further usage.

Other than lifestyle modifications, you can expect these treatments for getting pregnant:

- **Medication:** You might get medication for testosterone level and controlling insulin resistance.

- **Ovulation Induction:** It is medication for treating disorders of egg production. It usually starts from a lower dose and is increased through step-wise modification.

- **Laparoscopic Ovarian Drilling (LOD):** It is a minor surgical procedure conducted if ovulation induction does not work. The ovaries are drilled laparoscopically to restore ovulation. It has risks of causing permanent damage to ovaries or causing premature ovarian failure.

- **In Vitro Fertilization (IVF):** IVF is the preferred treatment. It can be the last stop for older or infertile women to use with limited options. If eligible, it has a 20-30% chance of working if all goes well.

You can use these treatment options with a doctor's recommendation. They can guide you toward a treatment that is specifically tailored for you.

6.3 Fertility Tracking and Ovulation Prediction

Understanding how ovulation takes place is a big concern for women trying to have a baby. There is a specific window in each month's cycle when a woman is most fertile, but contrary to popular belief, it does not necessarily occur on the same days of the cycle for every woman.

Since the beginning, we have been told that a menstrual cycle lasts 28 days, and on day 14, you start ovulation. But this is not the whole truth. A study shows that only 12% of women, in general, have a 28-day cycle. By extension, around 70% of women do not ovulate between 10 and 17 days into their cycles.

It is also possible for women to have changing ovulation dates with each cycle. This can make the tracking and prediction part more difficult. By tracking your own ovulation, you can learn about your body and its processes and use them to reach desired results.

Methods for Tracking Ovulation

There are three main categories in tracking the ovulation cycle. You can choose any one that seems most practical to you. They are as follows:

1. Fertility Awareness-Based Methods

These natural ways have been used for preventing pregnancy by many generations. They can also be used for tracking and making efforts to conceive. These methods include studying the days of the calendar and making predictions according to the period cycle (which can be inaccurate at times); using fingers to check the cervical mucus secretion (the more liquidity in secretion, the better ovulation); and checking basal body temperature for an increase in the body temperature right after waking up.

The body temperature technique is best for pinning down the days of ovulation only because it shows elevation in temperature after the 2-3 days of fertility window. Its a long process and can be used for months to find the exact fertility period.

2. Ovulation Predictor Kits (OPK)

Ovulation Predictor Kits are the most accurate method, with 99% accuracy. They detect the luteinizing hormone (LH) increase in the body 24-48 hours before ovulation. LH is responsible for triggering the ovaries to release the egg. The only downside is that OPKs cannot tell the level of LH surge.

Another thing to keep in mind is that sometimes the body can send a signal to the ovaries to release an egg through an LH increase, but the ovaries do not comprehend the message, resulting in the egg not being released.

3. Fertility Monitors

Fertility monitors are recommended because they are needed to identify the 3-day ovulation window and the LH surge. You can expect better results with fertility monitors, but they are an expensive option. The ovulation window detection is 88% accurate, while the LH surge detection is 99% accurate.

These methods are very easy to use. You can use any method as long as it is feasible for you. Natural fertility diets and lifestyle adjustments can also increase your chances of pregnancy.

Managing PCOS Symptoms

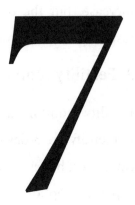

PCOS symptoms are bound to disturb your peace in one way or the other. When you start experiencing them, it is difficult to identify the cause, and many women blame other factors in their lives for causing the issues. For example, if you have acne on your skin, your first guess for its cause would not be PCOS. There could be many other factors in your mind like reaction to heat, dehydration, etc.

In the same way, we tend to ignore the causes and start treating the symptoms, hoping that we won't need to go to a doctor. If you are getting treatment for PCOS, there are some extra efforts you can make to keep its symptoms in check, too.

7.1 Skin and Hair Care Tips

PCOS can affect your hair and skin along with the reproductive system. There is no guarantee of who gets to experience which symptoms in PCOS. Here are some tips you can use to treat and manage acne, hair thinning, and hair growth excess (hirsutism):

Gentle Cleansing

Acne is the most common symptom of PCOS. Washing your face two times a day with a mild cleanser can help manage acne.

Harsh scrubs, excessive rubbing, and hard chemicals are all worse and should not be used. They can irritate the skin and worsen the acne.

Look for PCOS-friendly Products

When buying skincare products, it is necessary to opt for products labeled for sensitive or acne-prone skin. Benzoyl peroxide and salicylic acid are known ingredients for combating acne.

Non-comedogenic products are also suitable for acne-prone skin because they do not clog the pores.

Patch Test Technique

Before trying any new product, do a patch test. It will help you keep your skin away from any adverse reactions.

Regular Gentle Exfoliation

Gentle exfoliation once or twice a week can prevent acne flare-ups, remove dead skin cells, minimize breakouts, and smooth out the skin.

Hormonal Therapy

In extreme cases, a doctor can suggest you take hormonal therapy to improve hair and skin health. Birth control, anti-androgen, and other medications are all used for regulating the hormones.

Hair Removal Techniques

Waxing, threading, and laser treatment are all ways to combat hirsutism. They are used according to hair growth and preference. You can choose any approach that works best for you.

Making Hair Healthy Again

Use sulfate-free hair products to avoid hair thinning or hair loss. Add zinc and biotin to your diet to make hair follicles healthy. Tight hairstyles and heat styling products can also stress your hair.

You can also reduce your stress levels to make your hair and skin flourish. These are some of the best tips for keeping your hair and skin healthy. By taking time for self-care, you can work on your outlook and feel confident in your skin.

7.2 Menstrual Pain Management Techniques

Other than taking care of your skin and hair, managing the quite painful symptoms is also necessary. Every woman goes through menstrual pain once a month. But women with PCOS face worse symptoms than the rest. You can follow these techniques to counter the worst effects of menstruation:

NSAIDs

Non-steroidal anti-inflammatory drugs (NSAIDs) like Tylenol or Advil can relieve the pain, cramps, and other side effects that come with menstruation. They can reduce the production of enzymes that induce painful contractions.

Exercise and Yoga

Yoga and exercise are necessary for a healthy body and mind. Regular exercise can help regularize your periods and alleviate some adverse effects, as long as the workout is low-impact and easy to perform.

Heat Therapy

Hot water bottles, heating pads, or other warming techniques can also help relieve cramps and discomfort. Steam baths are also helpful for the same purpose.

Drink Lots of Water

Drinking plenty of water is always useful. It allows your body to function properly and feel energized. Keeping your water intake high can help the uterus contract less. It ensures normal uterine function and less pain from cramps. If possible, it is recommended to drink warm water. It can reduce stress, boost hydration, and improve digestion, among many other benefits.

Menstruation pain can be treated through some of these tested methods. By taking such measures, you can ensure a comfortable setting for yourself in your period days.

7.3 Coping with Mood Swings and Emotional Health

Mood swings are part of the equation for women. PCOS or not, you are bound to experience ups and downs in your emotional and mental state, bringing fluctuating hormones into the mix.

With PCOS, it is unlikely that you will experience the "traditional" mood swings that happen in Premenstrual

Syndrome or PMS. You may face unwanted feelings of hopelessness, grief, and others that stem from your low confidence, changing physique, and issues of hair and skin that are quite prevalent.

Once you start feeling less than others or listening to them for approval and happiness, you are more susceptible to feeling like an outsider. It increases the risk of deterioration in emotional and mental health with depression and anxiety.

> **Do You Know?**
>
> Women with PCOS are three times more at risk for having depression and anxiety.

Techniques for Reaching Emotional Well-Being

Emotional well-being is vital if you wish to stay true to yourself. There are some techniques that you can use to feel better and not let sadness or any other negative feeling take control over you. Some of them are as follows:

1. Focusing on the Moment

If you suddenly feel overwhelmed or off, it is better to take time and regroup yourself before participating with others or take a raincheck. Prioritize yourself above all else as a way of practicing self-care.

2. Note the Glaring Symptoms Down

Some PCOS symptoms are apparent, while others are not. It is better to write the symptoms as they appear to understand the progression and if they increase in intensity or disturb you more than usual.

Keeping a monthly or weekly log can allow you to stay aware and take measures at the right time.

3. Practice Mindfulness

It may seem unnecessary initially, but being mindful of your actions and behavior can open your eyes to new thought processes. We tend to cater to many negative or useless thoughts when not keeping ourselves in check. It ends with being mindful of all actions, whether big or small.

4. Breakfast Comes First

Drinking coffee as soon as you wake up is not a healthy practice. It is responsible for raising blood sugar levels. Always start your day with a balanced breakfast and maybe have coffee or tea afterward.

5. Check on Gluten and Dairy Items

They are not the best for everyone, nor are they the worst. Each person has different preferences and needs. You can try adding and subtracting dairy and gluten items from your diet as an experiment. Then, you can include or exclude them from your diet according to your gut feeling about them.

These are some of the techniques for managing PCOS while prioritizing emotional well-being. You should only practice the techniques that work best for you and give definite results.

Creating a Support System

8

A support system is a network of supporters and friends providing emotional and practical support. These people lend you an ear when you are agitated, sad, angry, or bursting with joy. You can expect yourself to have reliable support that lets you lean on it in the most trying circumstances.

This support network also reduces your anxiety and stress by helping you share challenging situations. Let's learn the importance and ways to find supportive communities you can join to stay successful.

8.1 Importance of a Support Network

Loneliness is never a solution. You may be independent and strong enough to endure any circumstance, but that does not mean you should have to.

Yes, you need a support group. You need to stay away from the negative influences. But it can only happen when you are ready to embrace yourself. If you are struggling in life because of PCOS or any other reason, you need to let people in. If you allow them to offer support in critical times, you are likelier to feel better soon enough.

Having a support group allows you to show resilience in tough times through support and enjoy the good times together. It also makes your mental, emotional, and physical health better.

Friends can provide guidance and help identify issues that you may not be able to crack yourself. This enhances the sense of security you get from finding comfort in their words.

A support group can also help you practice problem-solving skills that encourage you to take solution-oriented options rather than not facing the situation. They can also encourage you to stay strong in the face of adversity.

8.2 Finding Supportive Communities

Learning the art of making friends and acquaintances along the way is essential. It is by no means easy or something that can happen with the flick of a wrist. You need to put yourself on the line to make these resources.

No people who just happen to meet become friends instantly. You need to build trust, be open and forthcoming, respect others, and show your appreciation and thoughts so that others can open themselves up to you.

You can build a support system for yourself as follows:

1. Involving Family and Friends

You can involve your friends and family by actively seeking support from the ones you trust and adore. If they are not aware of PCOS and how it can affect you, it is better to educate them. You can ask them to match your pace and balance each other's needs and flaws simultaneously.

Many women ignore this crucial need because they feel ashamed or vulnerable, but you must face the situation head-on. Opening up with trusted, close friends and family can only comfort and calm you.

2. Finding and Joining Support Groups

Support groups are also great if you cannot use support from friends or family or if they seem inadequate. Many online and offline resources can help you counter the negative feelings about yourself with relatable stories and practical approaches that only a PCOS sufferer can share from experience.

You can make friends in these support groups or simply communicate your worries to receive advice from experienced people. They can guide you on how to not bottle up your feelings and make a real difference, even with PCOS.

3. Communicating with Healthcare Providers

Healthcare providers are your best friends when you must regain some semblance of everyday life. They can also be your most knowledgeable guides in the PCOS journey, telling you how to maximize the benefits and reduce the disadvantages of PCOS.

You can build a good working relationship with your doctor to maintain a healthy lifestyle that will benefit you in the long run. As long as you keep making regular appointments and follow their advice, nothing can go wrong from your end.

Having supportive people and communities around you can be a blessing in disguise. You can learn a lot from others– resilience, confidence, hope, or anything else. Keep uplifting yourself to stay on the right track, and let your supportive system help you lean on them in need.

Long-Term Management and Prevention

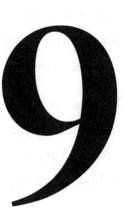

Managing stress, changing lifestyle, and following proper diet and exercise are all some of the ways that ensure a good life for PCOS patients. In terms of long-term management, there are a few other things you can do to get maximum benefit from the recommended practices.

You can use the techniques given ahead and any others you learn from learned doctors or researchers. Just make sure they are beneficial for you and allow you to get some benefits from them.

9.1 Keeping a Health Journal

A health journal is a simple yet effective way of documenting and tracking the conditions you face, their symptoms, and their progress. In a health journal, you can add categories for each day as follows:

- Diet Taken

- Exercise and Activity

- Sleep Quality

- Symptoms Experienced (with names and frequency)

- Any Unusual Symptoms/Behavior

- Notes (for recording extra information like weight gain/loss, treatments being conducted, etc.)

By keeping a detailed record of your health condition, you can stay informed about each change your body experiences. It is also a systematic way of keeping yourself aligned by not letting yourself deviate from the recommended practices if it is difficult for you to exercise self-control.

9.2 Regular Health Check-ups and Screenings

Having health check-ups and screenings every few months is a necessity, especially if you want to conceive in the future. You cannot lag behind if you want to live a full life. Always listen and consult with your doctor when there is anything that bothers you or seems unusual. The doctor might tell you to change medication, stop it, or offer other solutions that cater to your needs. But it can only happen when you are completely truthful with your doctor.

Stay on top of your health by closely monitoring your body's behaviors and imbalance levels. A few things that you should always be aware of are as follows:

- Glucose Tolerance
- Blood Pressure
- Cholesterol Level
- Triglycerides Level

9.3 Staying Motivated

Challenges and setbacks are part of the deal. You cannot expect yourself to only get good results. There may come a time when things don't go your way, but all you can do is stay charged and motivated to face anything that life throws at you.

You can stand against all odds by believing in your own capabilities, showing confidence and resilience, and taking practical measures. When you are feeling motivated, there is nothing you can't achieve.

You may start small by celebrating small victories and actions that bring you happiness before setting bigger goals and striving toward them.

As long as you are ready to fight, the battles will keep diminishing in front of your eyes. Your will to stay strong is the only long-term prevention and management technique you need in life. You cannot expect life to sail smoothly, but you can take measures to make it sail as smoothly as possible.

Conclusion

The PCOS Handbook is all about teaching and guiding you about PCOS. It is not a life-threatening condition, nor is it a benign or passive condition that leaves no effects. It is only about accepting reality and adjusting to it regardless of your feelings.

We make a lot of plans for our lives. Some are rooted in reality, while others are stuck in imagination. But there is one fact about plans: they change. Constantly. Take me for example. I wanted to be an artist when I grew up, but I changed my plan as soon as I realized how bad I was in the arts. It was so simple, and no one told me anything. Yet, I knew what had to be done. There was no point in pursuing something that held my fleeting attention rather than passion.

In the same way, I want you to choose. Choose life. Choose health. Choose going for the thing that will allow you to make PCOS your new normal.

Are you ready for it?

About the Author

W. Raymond is a gynecologist with 13 years of experience. She is a doctor, teacher, researcher, and activist who tries to motivate and guide her patients not to let their diagnosis define them. She has been working tirelessly to bring "The PCOS Handbook" for women who need to understand why having a life-long diagnosis is not the end of the world.